# Dash Diet Recipes For a Healthy Lifestyle

## Super Tasty Meals for a Healthy and Fit Life

Eleonore Barlow

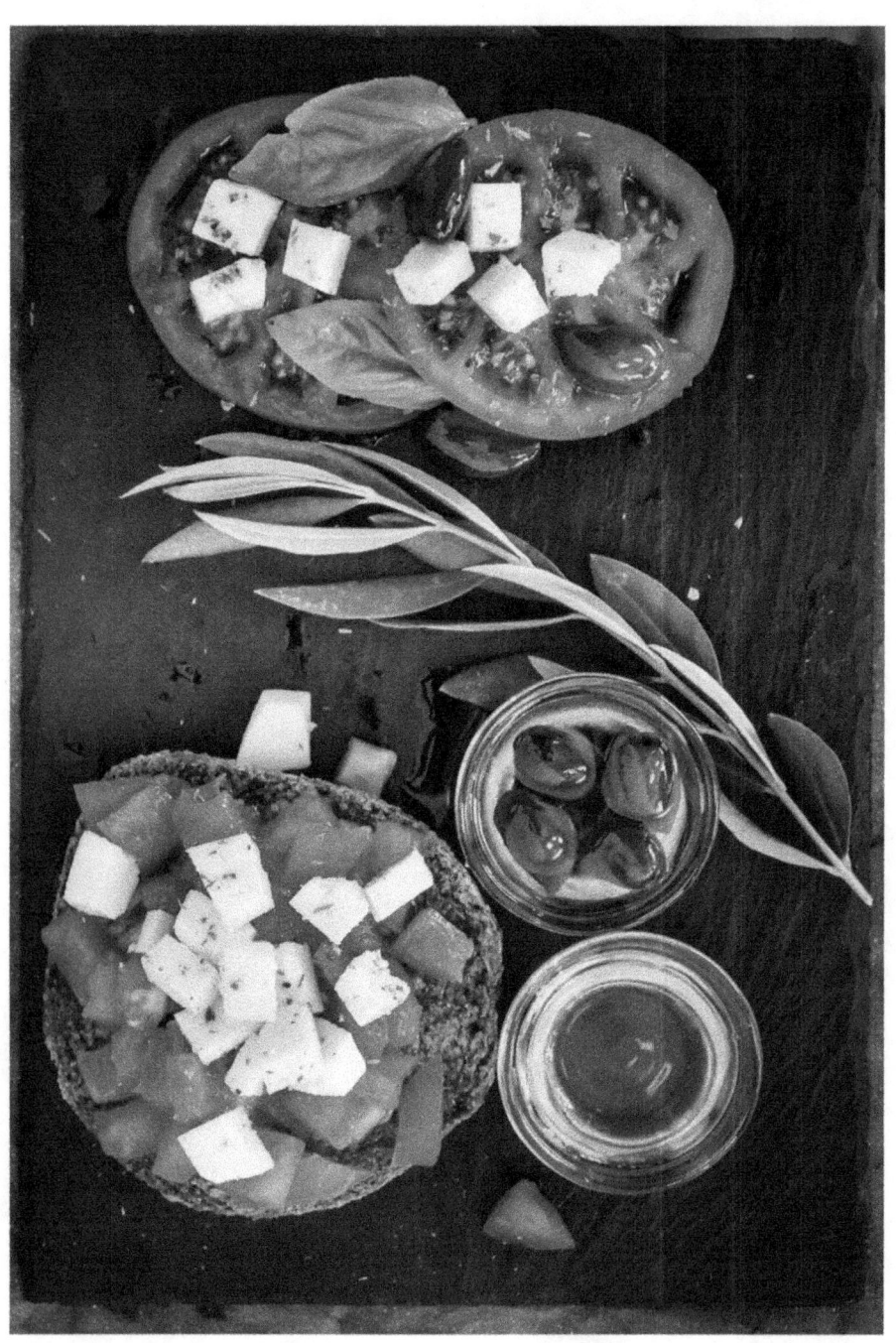

© Copyright 2021 - All rights reserved.

The content contained within this book may not be reproduced, duplicated or transmitted without direct written permission from the author or the publisher.
Under no circumstances will any blame or legal responsibility be held against the publisher, or author, for any damages, reparation, or monetary loss due to the information contained within this book. Either directly or indirectly.

**Legal Notice:**
This book is copyright protected. This book is only for personal use. You cannot amend, distribute, sell, use, quote or paraphrase any part, or the content within this book, without the consent of the author or publisher.

**Disclaimer Notice:**
Please note the information contained within this document is for educational and entertainment purposes only. All effort has been executed to present accurate, up to date, and reliable, complete information. No warranties of any kind are declared or implied. Readers acknowledge that the author is not engaging in the rendering of legal, financial, medical or professional advice. The content within this book has been derived from various sources. Please consult a licensed professional before attempting any techniques outlined in this book.
By reading this document, the reader agrees that under no circumstances is the author responsible for any losses, direct or indirect, which are incurred as a result of the use of information contained within this document, including, but not limited to, — errors, omissions, or inaccuracies.

# Table of Contents

- Olive Cherry Bites .................................................................. 6
- Roasted Herb Crackers ........................................................... 8
- Banana Steel Oats .................................................................. 10
- Swiss Chard Omelet ............................................................... 12
- Hearty Pineapple Oatmeal ...................................................... 14
- Zingy Onion and Thyme Crackers ........................................... 16
- Crunchy Flax and Almond Crackers ........................................ 18
- Duck with Cucumber and Carrots ........................................... 20
- Parmesan Baked Chicken ....................................................... 22
- Buffalo Chicken Lettuce Wraps ............................................... 25
- Crazy Japanese Potato and Beef Croquettes ........................... 27
- Spicy Chili Crackers ................................................................ 29
- Zucchini Zoodles with Chicken and Basil ................................ 31
- Tasty Roasted Broccoli ........................................................... 33
- The Almond Breaded Chicken Goodness ................................ 35
- South-Western Pork Chops .................................................... 37
- Ginger Zucchini Avocado Soup ............................................... 39
- Greek Lemon and Chicken Soup ............................................. 41
- Morning Peach ....................................................................... 43
- Garlic and Pumpkin Soup ....................................................... 45
- Butternut and Garlic Soup ...................................................... 47
- Minty Avocado Soup .............................................................. 49
- Celery, Cucumber and Zucchini Soup ..................................... 51
- Rosemary and Thyme Cucumber Soup ................................... 53
- Guacamole Soup .................................................................... 55
- Lemon and Garlic Scallops ..................................................... 57
- Walnut Encrusted Salmon ...................................................... 59

- Roasted Lemon Swordfish ............ 61
- Especial Glazed Salmon ............ 63
- Generous Stuffed Salmon Avocado ............ 66
- Insalata Capricciosa ............ 68
- Oopsie sandwich (keto) ............ 70
- Keto (gluten-free) poffertjes ............ 72
- Frittata with Chanterelles ............ 74
- The Refreshing Nutter ............ 77
- Elegant Cranberry Muffins ............ 79
- Apple and Almond Muffins ............ 82
- Stylish Chocolate Parfait ............ 84
- Supreme Matcha Bomb ............ 86
- Mesmerizing Avocado and Chocolate Pudding ............ 88
- Hearty Pineapple Pudding ............ 90
- The Mean Green Smoothie ............ 92
- Mint Flavored Pear Smoothie ............ 94
- Chilled Watermelon Smoothie ............ 95
- Banana Ginger Medley ............ 97
- Banana and Almond Flax Glass ............ 98
- Protein 2gSpicy Wasabi Mayonnaise ............ 99
- Mediterranean Kale Dish ............ 101
- Delicious Garlic Tomatoes ............ 103
- Mashed Celeriac ............ 105

# Olive Cherry Bites

Serving: 30

Prep Time: 15 minutes

Cook Time: Nil

## Ingredients:

24 cherry tomatoes, halved

24 black olives, pitted

24 feta cheese cubes

24 toothpick/decorative skewers

## How To:

1. Use a toothpick or skewer and thread feta cheese, black olives, cherry tomato halves therein order.

2. Repeat until all the ingredients are used.

3. Arrange during a serving platter.

4. Serve and enjoy!

**Nutrition (Per Serving)**

Calories: 57

Fat: 5g

Carbohydrates: 2g

Protein: 2g

# Roasted Herb Crackers

Serving: 75 Crackers

Prep Time: 10 minutes

Cook Time: 120 minutes

**Ingredients:**

¼ cup avocado oil

10 celery sticks

1 sprig fresh rosemary, stem discarded

2 sprigs fresh thyme, stems discarded

2 tablespoons apple cider vinegar

1 teaspoon Himalayan sunflower seeds

3 cups ground flaxseeds

**How To:**

1. Preheat your oven to 225 degrees F.
2. Line a baking sheet with parchment paper and keep it on the side.

3.   Add oil, herbs, celery, vinegar, sunflower seeds to a kitchen appliance and pulse until you've got a good mixture.

4.   Add flax and puree.

5.   Let it sit for 2-3 minutes.

6.   Transfer batter to your prepared baking sheet and spread evenly, dig cracker shapes.

7.   Bake for hour , flip and bake for hour more.

8.   Enjoy!

**Nutrition (Per Serving)**

Calories: 34

Fat: 5g

Carbohydrates: 1g

Protein: 1.3g

# Banana Steel Oats

Serving: 3

Prep Time: 10 minutes

Cook Time: 15 minutes

## Ingredients:

1 small banana

1 cup almond milk

¼ teaspoon cinnamon, ground

½ cup rolled oats

1 tablespoon honey

## How To:

1. Take a saucepan and add half the banana, whisk in almond milk, ground cinnamon.

2. Season with sunflower seeds.

3. Stir until the banana is mashed well, bring the mixture to a boil and stir in oats.

4. Reduce heat to medium-low and simmer for 5-7 minutes until the oats are tender.

5. Dice the remaining half banana and placed on the highest of the oatmeal.

6. Enjoy!

**Nutrition (Per Serving)**

Calories: 358

Fat: 6g

Carbohydrates: 76g

Protein: 7g

# Swiss Chard Omelet

Serving: 2

Prep Time: 5 minutes

Cook Time: 5 minutes

**Ingredients:**

2 eggs, lightly beaten

2 cups Swiss chard, sliced

1 tablespoon almond butter

½ teaspoon sunflower seeds Fresh pepper

**How To:**

1. Take a non-stick frypan and place it over medium-low heat.

2. Once the almond butter melts, add Swiss chard and stir-cook for two minutes.

3. Pour the eggs into the pan and gently stir them into Swiss chard.

4. Season with garlic sunflower seeds and pepper.

5. Cook for two minutes.

6. Serve and enjoy!

**Nutrition (Per Serving)**

Calories: 260

Fat: 21g

Carbohydrates: 4g

Protein: 14g

# Hearty Pineapple Oatmeal

Serving: 5

Prep Time: 10 minutes

Cook Time: 4-8 hours

**Ingredients:**

1 cup steel-cut oats

4 cups unsweetened almond milk

2 medium apples, sliced

1 teaspoon coconut oil

1 teaspoon cinnamon

¼ teaspoon nutmeg

2 tablespoons maple syrup, unsweetened A drizzle of lemon juice

**How To:**

1. Add listed ingredients to a pan and blend well.
2. Cook on very low flame for 8 hours/or on high flame for 4 hours.

3. Gently stir.

4. Add your required toppings.

5. Serve and enjoy!

6. Store within the fridge for later use; confirm to feature a splash of almond milk after re-heating for added flavor.

**Nutrition (Per Serving)**

Calories: 180

Fat: 5g

Carbohydrates: 31g

Protein: 5g

# Zingy Onion and Thyme Crackers

Serving: 75 crackers

Prep Time: 15 minutes

Cooking Time: 120 minutes

## Ingredients:

1 garlic clove, minced

1 cup sweet onion, coarsely chopped

2 teaspoons fresh thyme leaves

¼ cup avocado oil

¼ teaspoon garlic powder

Freshly ground black pepper

¼ cup sunflower seeds

1 ½ cups roughly ground flax seeds

## How To:

1. Preheat your oven to 225 degrees F.

2.   Line two baking sheets with parchment paper and keep it on the side.

3.   Add garlic, onion, thyme, oil, sunflower seeds, and pepper to a kitchen appliance.

4.   Add sunflower and flax seeds, pulse until pureed.

5.   Transfer the batter to prepared baking sheets and spread evenly, dig crackers

6.   Bake for hour.

7.   Remove parchment paper and flip crackers, bake for an additional hour.

8.   If crackers are thick, it'll take longer.

9.   Remove from oven and allow them to cool.

10.   Enjoy!

**Nutrition (Per Serving)**

Total Carbs: 0.8g

Fiber: 0.2g

Protein: 0.4g

Fat: 2.7g

# Crunchy Flax and Almond Crackers

Serving: 20-24 crackers

Prep Time: 15 minutes

Cooking Time: 60 minutes

**Ingredients:**

½ cup ground flaxseeds

½ cup almond flour

1 tablespoon coconut flour

2 tablespoons shelled hemp seeds

¼ teaspoon sunflower seeds

1 egg white

2 tablespoons unsalted almond butter, melted

**How To:**

1. Preheat your oven to 300 degrees F.

2. Line a baking sheet with parchment paper, keep it on the side.

3. Add flax, almond, coconut flour, hemp seed, seeds to a bowl and blend.

4. Add albumen and melted almond butter, mix until combined.

5. Transfer dough to a sheet of parchment paper and canopy with another sheet of paper.

6. Roll out dough.

7. dig crackers and bake for hour.

8. allow them to cool and enjoy!

**Nutrition (Per Serving)**

Total Carbs: 1.2

Fiber: 1g

Protein: 2g

Fat: 6g

# Duck with Cucumber and Carrots

Serving: 8

Prep Time: 10 minutes

Cook Time: 40 minutes

**Ingredients:**

1 duck, cut up into medium pieces

1 chopped cucumber, chopped

1 tablespoon low sodium vegetable stock

2 carrots, chopped

2 cups of water

Black pepper as needed

1-inch ginger piece, grated

**How To:**

1. Add duck pieces to your Instant Pot.

2. Add cucumber, stock, carrots, water, ginger, pepper and stir.

3. Lock up the lid and cook on low for 40 minutes.

4. Release the pressure naturally.

5. Serve and enjoy!

**Nutrition (Per Serving)**

Calories: 206

Fats: 7g

Carbs: 28g

Protein: 16g

# Parmesan Baked Chicken

Serving: 2

Prep Time: 5 minutes

Cook Time: 20 minutes

**Ingredients:**

2 tablespoons ghee

2 boneless chicken breasts, skinless

Pink sunflower seeds

Freshly ground black pepper

½ cup mayonnaise, low fat

¼ cup parmesan cheese, grated

1 tablespoon dried Italian seasoning, low fat, low sodium ¼ cup crushed pork rinds

**How To:**

1. Preheat your oven to 425 degrees F.
2. Take an outsized baking dish and coat with ghee.

3. Pat chicken breasts dry and wrap with a towel.

4. Season with sunflower seeds and pepper.

5. Place in baking dish.

6. Take a little bowl and add mayonnaise, parmesan cheese, Italian seasoning.

7. Slather mayo mix evenly over pigeon breast.

8. Sprinkle crushed pork rinds on top.

9. Bake for 20 minutes until topping is browned.

10. Serve and enjoy!

**Nutrition (Per Serving)**

Calories: 850

Fat: 67g

Carbohydrates: 2g

Protein: 60g

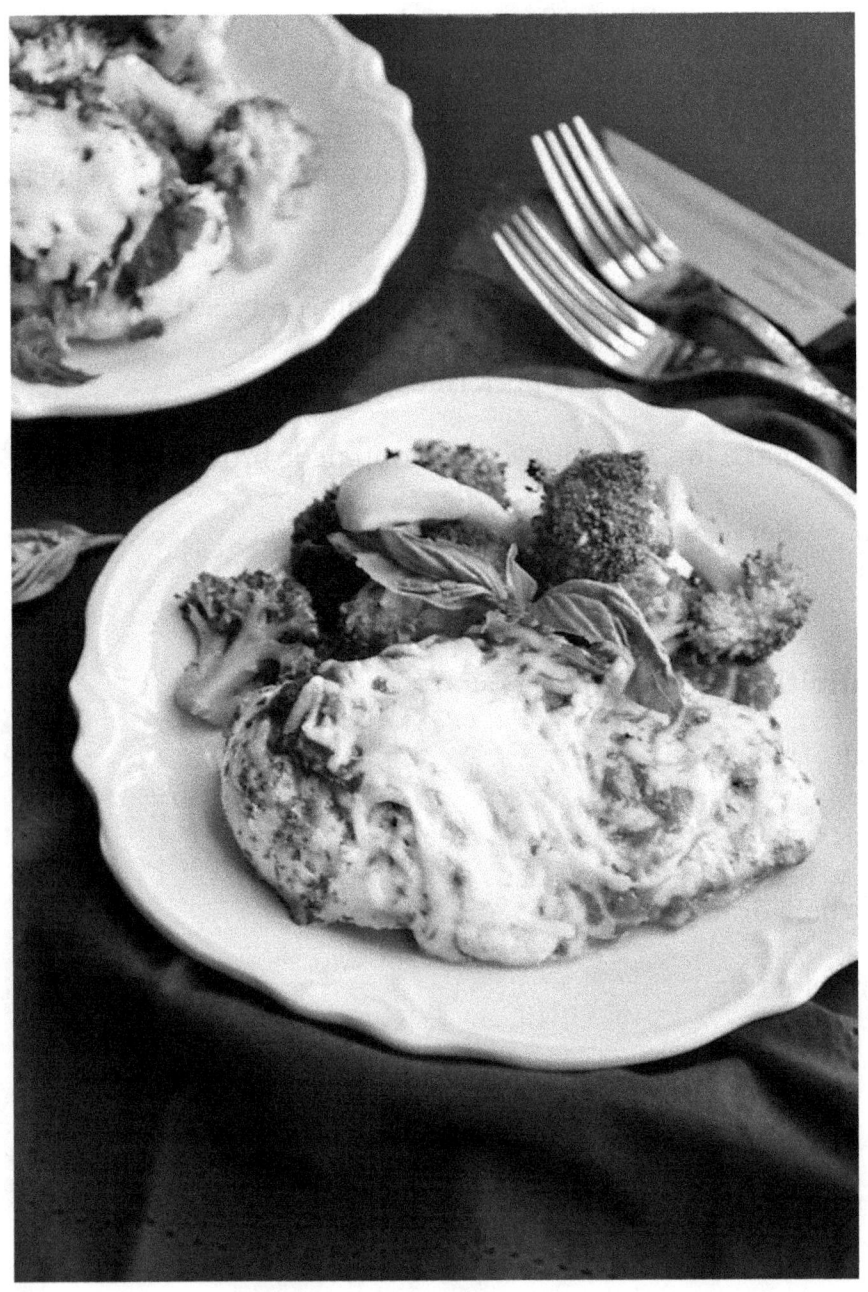

# Buffalo Chicken Lettuce Wraps

Serving: 2

Prep Time: 35 minutes

Cook Time: 10 minutes

**Ingredients:**

3 chicken breasts, boneless and cubed

20 slices of almond butter lettuce leaves ¾ cup cherry tomatoes halved

1 avocado, chopped

¼ cup green onions, diced

½ cup ranch dressing

¾ cup hot sauce

**How To:**

1. Take a bowl and add chicken cubes and sauce , mix.
2. Place within the fridge and let it marinate for half-hour .
3. Preheat your oven to 400 degrees F.

4. Place coated chicken on a cookie pan and bake for 9 minutes.

5. Assemble lettuce serving cups with equal amounts of lettuce, green onions, tomatoes, ranch dressing, and cubed chicken.

6. Serve and enjoy!

**Nutrition (Per Serving)**

Calories: 106

Fat: 6g

Net Carbohydrates: 2g

Protein: 5g

# Crazy Japanese Potato and Beef Croquettes

Serving: 10

Prep Time: 10 minutes

Cook Time: 20 minutes

**Ingredients:**

3 medium russet potatoes, peeled and chopped

1 tablespoon almond butter

1 tablespoon vegetable oil

3 onions, diced

¾ pound ground beef

4 teaspoons light coconut aminos

All-purpose flour for coating

2 eggs, beaten

Panko bread crumbs for coating

½ cup oil, frying

**How To:**

1. Take a saucepan and place it over medium-high heat; add potatoes and sunflower seeds water, boil for 16 minutes.

2. Remove water and put potatoes in another bowl, add almond butter and mash the potatoes.

3. Take a frypan and place it over medium heat, add 1 tablespoon oil and let it heat up.

4. Add onions and fry until tender.

5. Add coconut aminos to beef to onions.

6. Keep frying until beef is browned.

7. Mix the meat with the potatoes evenly.

8. Take another frypan and place it over medium heat; add half a cup of oil.

9. Form croquettes using the potato mixture and coat them with flour, then eggs and eventually breadcrumbs.

10. Fry patties until golden on all sides.

11. Enjoy!

## Nutrition (Per Serving)

Calories: 239
Fat: 4g
Carbohydrates: 20g
Protein: 10g

# Spicy Chili Crackers

Serving: 30 crackers

Prep Time: 15 minutes

Cooking Time: 60 minutes

**Ingredients:**

¾ cup almond flour

¼ cup coconut four

¼ cup coconut flour

½ teaspoon paprika

½ teaspoon cumin

1 ½ teaspoons chili pepper spice

1 teaspoon onion powder

½ teaspoon sunflower seeds

1 whole egg

¼ cup unsalted almond butter

## How To:

1. Preheat your oven to 350 degrees F.

2. Line a baking sheet with parchment paper and keep it on the side.

3. Add ingredients to your kitchen appliance and pulse until you've got a pleasant dough.

4. Divide dough into two equal parts.

5. Place one ball on a sheet of parchment paper and canopy with another sheet; roll it out.

6. dig crackers and repeat with the opposite ball.

7. Transfer the prepped dough to a baking tray and bake for 8-10 minutes.

8. Remove from oven and serve.

9. Enjoy!

## Nutrition (Per Serving)

Total Carbs: 2.8g

Fiber: 1g

Protein: 1.6g

Fat: 4.1g

# Zucchini Zoodles with Chicken and Basil

Serving: 2

Prep Time: 10 minutes

Cook Time: 10 minutes

**Ingredients:**

2 chicken fillets, cubed

2 tablespoons ghee

1-pound tomatoes, diced

½ cup basil, chopped

¼ cup coconut almond milk

1 garlic clove, peeled, minced

1 zucchini, shredded

**How To:**

1. Sauté cubed chicken in ghee until not pink.
2. Add tomatoes and season with sunflower seeds.
3. Simmer and reduce the liquid.

4. Prepare your zucchini Zoodles by shredding zucchini during a kitchen appliance.

5. Add basil, garlic, coconut almond milk to chicken and cook for a couple of minutes.

6. Add half the zucchini Zoodles to a bowl and top with creamy tomato basil chicken.

7. Enjoy!

## Nutrition (Per Serving)

Calories: 540

Fat: 27g

Carbohydrates: 13g

Protein: 59g

# Tasty Roasted Broccoli

Serving: 4

Prep Time: 5 minutes

Cook Time: 20 minutes

**Ingredients:**

4 cups broccoli florets

1 tablespoon olive oil

Sunflower seeds and pepper to taste

**How To:**

1. Pre-heat your oven to 400 degrees F.
2. Add broccoli during a zip bag alongside oil and shake until coated.
3. Add seasoning and shake again.
4. Spread broccoli out on baking sheet, bake for 20 minutes.
5. Let it cool and serve.
6. Enjoy!

**Nutrition (Per Serving)**

Calories: 62

Fat: 4g

Carbohydrates: 4g

Protein: 4g

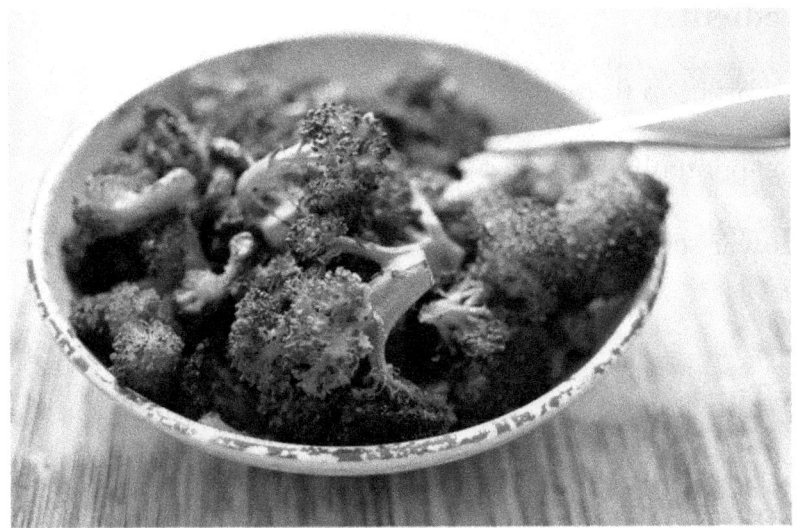

# The Almond Breaded Chicken Goodness

Serving: 3

Prep Time: 15 minutes

Cook Time: 15 minutes

**Ingredients:**

2 large chicken breasts, boneless and skinless 1/3 cup lemon juice

1 ½ cups seasoned almond meal

2 tablespoons coconut oil

Lemon pepper, to taste

Parsley for decoration

**How To:**

1. Slice pigeon breast in half.

2. Pound out each half until ¼ inch thick.

3. Take a pan and place it over medium heat, add oil and warmth it up.

4.  Dip each pigeon breast slice through juice and let it sit for two minutes.

5.  Turnover and therefore the let the opposite side sit for two minutes also.

6.  Transfer to almond meal and coat each side.

7.  Add coated chicken to the oil and fry for 4 minutes per side, ensuring to sprinkle lemon pepper liberally.

8.  Transfer to a paper lined sheet and repeat until all chicken are fried.

9.  Garnish with parsley and enjoy!

**Nutrition (Per Serving)**

Calories: 325

Fat: 24g

Carbohydrates: 3g

Protein: 16g

# South-Western Pork Chops

Serving: 4

Prep Time: 10 minutes

Cook Time: 15 minutes

Smart Points: 3

**Ingredients:**

Cooking spray as needed 4-ounce pork loin chop, boneless and fat rimmed 1/3 cup salsa

2 tablespoons fresh lime juice

¼ cup fresh cilantro, chopped

**How To:**

1. Take an outsized sized non-stick skillet and spray it with cooking spray.

2. Heat until hot over high heat.

3. Press the chops together with your palm to flatten them slightly.

4. Add them to the skillet and cook on 1 minute for every side until they're nicely browned.

5. Lower the warmth to medium-low.

6. Combine the salsa and juice.

7. Pour the combination over the chops.

8. Simmer uncovered for about 8 minutes until the chops are perfectly done.

9. If needed, sprinkle some cilantro on top.

10. Serve!

**Nutrition (Per Serving)**

Calorie: 184

Fat: 4g

Carbohydrates: 4g

Protein: 0.5g

# Ginger Zucchini Avocado Soup

Serving: 3

Prep Time: 7 minutes

Cook Time: 25 minutes

**Ingredients:**

1 red bell pepper, chopped

1 big avocado

1 teaspoon ginger, grated

Pepper as needed

2 tablespoons avocado oil

4 scallions, chopped

1 tablespoon lemon juice

29 ounces vegetable stock

1 garlic clove, minced

2 zucchini, chopped

1 cup water

**How To:**

1. Take a pan and place over medium heat, add onion and fry for 3 minutes.

2. Stir in ginger, garlic and cook for 1 minute.

3. Mix in seasoning, zucchini stock, water and boil for 10 minutes.

4. Remove soup from fire and let it sit, blend in avocado and blend using an immersion blender.

5. Heat over low heat for a short time .

6. Adjust your seasoning and add juice , bell pepper.

7. Serve and enjoy!

**Nutrition (Per Serving)**

Calories: 155

Fat: 11g

Carbohydrates: 10g

Protein: 7g

# Greek Lemon and Chicken Soup

Serving: 4

Prep Time: 15 minutes

Cook Time: 30 minutes

**Ingredients:**

2 cups cooked chicken, chopped

2 medium carrots, chopped

½ cup onion, chopped ¼ cup lemon juice 1 clove garlic, minced

1 can cream of chicken soup, fat-free and low sodium

2 cans chicken broth, fat-free

¼ teaspoon ground black pepper

2/3 cup long-grain rice

2 tablespoons parsley, snipped

**How To:**

1. Add all of the listed ingredients to a pot (except rice and parsley).

2. Season with sunflower seeds and pepper.

3. Bring the combination to a overboil medium-high heat.

4. Stir in rice and set heat to medium.

5. Simmer for 20 minutes until rice is tender.

6. Garnish parsley and enjoy!

**Nutrition (Per Serving)**

Calories: 582

Fat: 33g

Carbohydrates: 35g

Protein: 32g

# Morning Peach

Serving: 4

Prep Time: 10 minutes

Cook Time: 5 minutes

**Ingredients:**

6 small peaches, cored and cut into wedges ¼ cup coconut sugar

2 tablespoons almond butter

¼ teaspoon almond extract

**How To:**

1. Take alittle pan and add peaches, sugar, butter and flavor.
2. Toss well.
3. Cook over medium-high heat for five minutes, divide the combination into bowls and serve.
4. Enjoy!

**Nutrition (Per Serving)**

Calories: 198

Fat: 2g

Carbohydrates: 11g

Protein: 8g

# Garlic and Pumpkin Soup

Serving: 4

Prep Time: 10 minutes

Cook Time: 5 hours

**Ingredients:**

1-pound pumpkin chunks

1 onion, diced

2 cups vegetable stock

1 2/3 cups coconut cream

½ stick almond butter

1 teaspoon garlic, crushed

1 teaspoon ginger, crushed

Pepper to taste

**How To:**

1. Add all the ingredients into your Slow Cooker.
2. Cook for 4-6 hours on high.

3. Puree the soup by using an immersion blender.

4. Serve and enjoy!

**Nutrition (Per Serving)**

Calories: 235

Fat: 21g

Carbohydrates: 11g

Protein: 2g

# Butternut and Garlic Soup

Serving: 4

Prep Time: 5 minutes

Cook Time: 35 minutes

## Ingredients:

4 cups butternut squash, cubed

4 cups vegetable broth, stock

½ cup low fat cream

2 garlic cloves, chopped

Pepper to taste

## How To:

1. Add butternut squash, garlic cloves, broth, salt and pepper during a large pot.

2. Place the pot over medium heat and canopy with the lid.

3. Bring back boil then reduce the temperature.

4. Let it simmer for 30-35 minutes.[MOU7]

5. Blend the soup for 1-2 minutes until you get a smooth mixture.

6. Stir the cream through the soup.

7. Serve and enjoy!

**Nutrition (Per Serving)**

Calories: 180

Fat: 14g

Carbohydrates: 21g

Protein: 3g

# Minty Avocado Soup

Serving: 4

Prep Time: 10 minutes + Chill time

Cook Time: nil

**Ingredients:**

1 avocado, ripe

1 cup coconut almond milk, chilled

2 romaine lettuce leaves

20 mint leaves, fresh

1 tablespoon lime juice

Sunflower seeds, to taste

**How To:**

1. Activate your slow cooker and add all the ingredients into it.

2. Mix them during a kitchen appliance.

3. Make a smooth mixture.

4. Let it chill for 10 minutes.

5. Serve and enjoy!

**Nutrition (Per Serving)**

Calories: 280

Fat: 26g

Carbohydrates: 12g

Protein: 4g

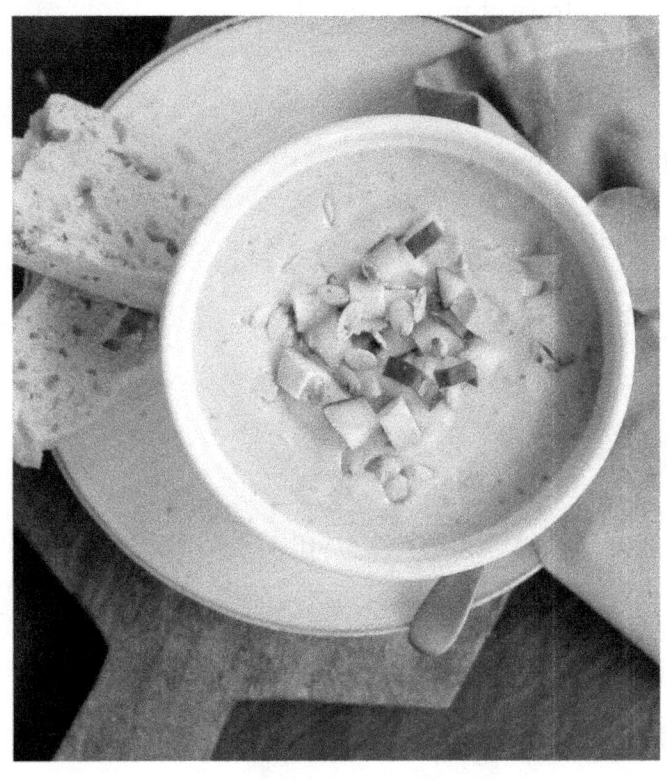

# Celery, Cucumber and Zucchini Soup

Serving: 2

Prep Time: 10 minutes + Chill time

Cook Time: nil

**Ingredients:**

3 celery stalks, chopped

7 ounces cucumber, cubed

1 tablespoon olive oil

2/5 cup fresh cream, 30%, low fat

1 red bell pepper, chopped

1 tablespoon dill, chopped

10 ½ ounces zucchini, cubed

Sunflower seeds and pepper, to taste

**How To:**

1. Put the vegetables during a juicer and juice.

2. Then mix within the vegetable oil and fresh cream.

3. Season with sauce and pepper.

4. Garnish with dill.

5. Serve it chilled and enjoy!

**Nutrition (Per Serving)**

Calories: 325

Fat: 32g

Carbohydrates: 10g

Protein: 4g

# Rosemary and Thyme Cucumber Soup

Serving: 3

Prep Time: 10 minutes + Chill time

Cook Time: nil

**Ingredients:**

4 cups vegetable broth

1 teaspoon thyme, freshly chopped

1 teaspoon rosemary, freshly chopped

2 cucumbers, sliced1 cup low fat cream

1 pinch of sunflower seeds

**How To:**

1. Take an outsized bowl and add all the ingredients.
2. Whisk well.
3. Blend until smooth by using an immersion blender.
4. Let it chill for 1 hour.
5. Serve and enjoy!

**Nutrition (Per Serving)**

Calories: 111

Fat: 8g

Carbohydrates: 4g

Protein: 5g

# Guacamole Soup

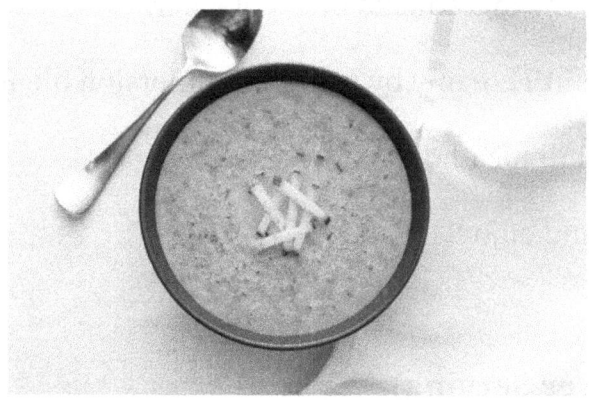

Serving: 3

Prep Time: 10 minute + Chill time

Cook Time: nil

**Ingredients:**

3 cups vegetable broth 2 ripe avocados, pitted ½ cup cilantro, freshly chopped

1 tomato, chopped

½ cup low fat cream

Sunflower seeds & black pepper, to taste

**How To:**

1. Add all the ingredients into a blender.

2. Blend until creamy by using an immersion blender.

3. Let it chill for 1 hour.

4. Serve and enjoy!

**Nutrition (Per Serving)**

Calories: 289

Fat: 26g

Carbohydrates: 5g

Protein: 10g

# Lemon and Garlic Scallops

Serving: 4

Prep Time: 10 minutes

Cook Time: 5 minutes

**Ingredients:**

1 tablespoon olive oil

¼ pounds dried scallops

tablespoons all-purpose flour

¼ teaspoon sunflower seeds

4-5 garlic cloves, minced

1 scallion, chopped

1 pinch of ground sage

lemon juice

tablespoons parsley, chopped

**Direction**

1. Take a non-stick skillet and place over medium-high heat.

2. Add oil and permit the oil to heat up.

3. Take a medium sized bowl and add scallops alongside sunflower seeds and flour.

4. Place the scallops within the skillet and add scallions, garlic, and sage.

5. Sauté for 3-4 minutes until they show an opaque texture.

6. Stir in juice and parsley.

7. Remove heat and serve hot!

**Nutrition (Per Serving)**

Calories: 151

Fat: 4g

Carbohydrates: 10g

Protein: 18g

# Walnut Encrusted Salmon

Serving: 34

Prep Time: 10 minutes

Cook Time: 14 minutes

**Ingredients:**

½ cup walnuts

tablespoons stevia

½ tablespoon Dijon mustard

¼ teaspoon dill

salmon fillets (3 ounces each)

1 tablespoon olive oil

Sunflower seeds and pepper to taste

**How To:**

1. Pre-heat your oven to 350 degrees F.

2. Add walnuts, mustard, stevia to kitchen appliance and process until your required consistency is achieved.

3. Take a frypan and place it over medium heat.

4. Add oil and let it heat up.

5. Add salmon and sear for 3 minutes.

6. Add walnut mix and coat well.

7. Transfer coated salmon to baking sheet, bake in oven for 8 minutes.

8. Serve and enjoy!

## Nutrition (Per Serving)

Calories: 373

Fat: 43g

Carbohydrates: 4g

Protein: 20g

# Roasted Lemon Swordfish

Serving: 4

Prep Time: 10 minutes

Cook Time: 70-80 minutes

**Ingredients:**

¼ cup parsley, chopped

½ teaspoon garlic, chopped

½ teaspoon canola oil

swordfish fillets, 6 ounces each

¼ teaspoon sunflower seeds

tablespoon sugar

lemons, quartered and seeds removed

**How To:**

1. Preheat your oven to 375 degrees F.

2. Take a small-sized bowl and add sugar, sunflower seeds, lemon wedges.

3. Toss well to coat them.

4. Take a shallow baking dish and add lemons, cover with aluminum foil.

5. Roast for about hour until lemons are tender and browned (Slightly).

6. Heat your grill and place the rack about 4 inches far away from the source of warmth.

7. Take a baking pan and coat it with cooking spray.

8. Transfer fish fillets to the pan and brush with oil on top spread garlic on top.

9. Grill for about 5 minutes all sides until fillet turns opaque.

10. Transfer fish to a serving platter, squeeze roasted lemon on top.

11. Sprinkle parsley, serve with a lemon wedge on the side.

12. Enjoy!

## Nutrition (Per Serving)

Calories: 280

Fat: 12g

Net Carbohydrates: 4g

Protein: 34g

# Especial Glazed Salmon

Serving: 4

Prep Time: 45 minutes

Cook Time: 10 minutes

**Ingredients:**

Pieces of salmon fillets, 5 ounces each

tablespoons coconut aminos

Teaspoon olive oil

2 teaspoons ginger, minced

teaspoons garlic, minced

2 tablespoons sugar-free ketchup

tablespoons dry white wine

2 tablespoons red boat fish sauce, low sodium

**How To:**

1. Take a bowl and blend in coconut aminos, garlic, ginger, fish sauce and blend.

2. Add salmon and let it marinate for 15-20 minutes.

3. Take a skillet/pan and place it over medium heat.

4. Add oil and let it heat up.

5. Add salmon fillets and cook on high heat for 3-4 minutes per side.

6. Remove dish once crispy.

7. Add sauce and wine.

8. Simmer for five minutes on low heat.

9. Return salmon to the glaze and flip until each side are glazed.

10. Serve and enjoy!

**Nutrition (Per Serving)**

Calories: 372

Fat: 24g

Carbohydrates: 3g

Protein: 35g

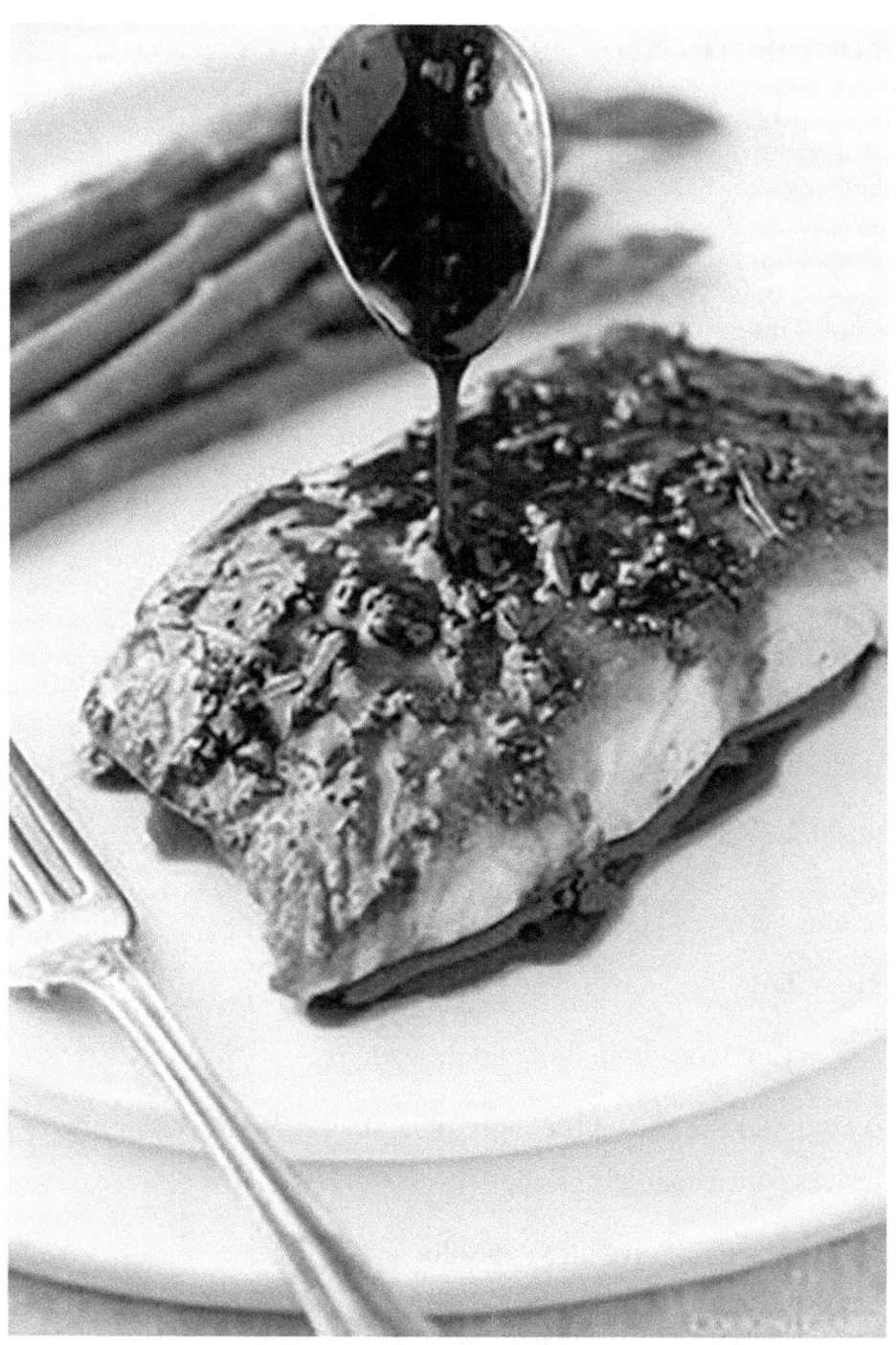

# Generous Stuffed Salmon Avocado

Serving: 2

Prep Time: 10 minutes

Cook Time: 30 minutes

**Ingredients:**

ripe organic avocado

ounces wild caught smoked salmon

ounce cashew cheese

tablespoons extra virgin olive oil

Sunflower seeds as needed

**How To:**

1. Cut avocado in half and deseed.
2. Add the rest of the ingredients to a food processor and process until coarsely chopped.
3. Place mixture into avocado.
4. Serve and enjoy!

**Nutrition (Per Serving)**

Calories: 525

Fat: 48g

Carbohydrates: 4g

Protein: 19g

# Insalata Capricciosa

## Nutrition

Calories: 551 kcal | Gross carbohydrates: 9 g | Protein: 28 g | Fats: 46 g | Fiber: 3 g | Net carbohydrates: 6 g | Macro fats: 58 % | Macro proteins: 35 % | Macro carbohydrates: 8 %

Time: 15 minutes

## Ingredients

2 eggs

2 tomatoes around 200 grams

100 grams of mixed lettuce or iceberg lettuce

60 grams of black olives, preferably in olive oil

100 grams of mozzarella

100 grams of tuna in water or olive oil

pepper and salt

50 ml extra virgin olive oil

15 ml of lemon juice

## Instructions

1. Bring a saucepan of water to the boil. Once the water boils, carefully lay the eggs in it. Bring the water back to the boil and boil the eggs for 8 minutes. Then place the pan under the cold tap so that the eggs cool sufficiently to allow them to peel.

2.   Wash the tomatoes, pat them dry with kitchen paper and cut into slices.

3.   Drain the tuna well and place it on top of the lettuce.

4.   Also, divide the tomato and olives slices over the lettuce and also cut the boiled eggs into slices. Put it on the lettuce too.

5.   Season the salad with salt and pepper. Make a vinaigrette by mixing the olive oil well with the lemon juice in a cup. Use a teaspoon to distribute the vinaigrette on the plates.

# Oopsie sandwich (keto)

## Nutrition

Calories: 84 kcal | Gross carbohydrates: 2 g | Protein: 4 g | Fats: 7 g | Fiber: 1g | Net carbohydrates: 1 g | Macro fats: 58 % | Macro proteins: 33 % | Macro carbohydrates: 8 %

Total time: 30 minutes

## Ingredients

2 eggs

75 grams of cream cheese

1 teaspoon of psyllium

0.5 teaspoon baking powder

pinch of salt

## Instructions

1. Preheat the oven to 150° Celsius and ensure that the eggs are at room temperature. When the eggs come out of the refrigerator, place them in a bowl of lukewarm tap water for 10-15 minutes.

2. Split the eggs. Put the egg whites in a cup for a hand blender and the egg yolks in another bowl.

3. Mix the egg yolks with the cream cheese, the psyllium and the baking powder with a whisk or a fork. Let this batter rest for 5 minutes so that the baking powder and psyllium can work.

4.     Beat the egg whites with a pinch of salt. The proteins must be so stiff that if you hold the cup upside down, they will not move.

5.     Carefully scoop the egg whites through the egg yolk-cream cheese mixture. The mixture must become nicely airy.

6.     Put a sheet of baking paper on an oven plate and make 8 heaps of batter on the baking sheet.

7.     Bake in 25 minutes at 150° Celsius. The sandwiches must be beautifully golden brown.

# Keto (gluten-free) poffertjes

## Nutrition

Calories: 700 kcal | Gross carbohydrates: 8 g | Protein: 27 g | Fats: 63 g |Fiber: 1 g | Net carbohydrates: 7 g | Macro fats: 65 % | Macro proteins: 28 % |Macro carbohydrates: 7 %

Total time: 40 minutes

## Ingredients

Keto poffertjes

4 eggs

250 grams of ricotta

1 tablespoon psyllium, for example, Livinggreens psyllium fibers

0.5 teaspoon baking powder

0.25 teaspoon vanilla extract

2 tablespoons of mild olive oil

Whipped cream

200 ml whipped cream

0.5 teaspoon vanilla extract

## Instructions

1. Allow the eggs to reach room temperature by removing them from the fridge 15 minutes in advance or by placing them in lukewarm tap water for 5 minutes.

2. If you have made your own ricotta, use a hand blender or hand blender until there are no / few lumps. If you have ricotta from the store this is not necessary.

3. Now add the ricotta, the baking powder (optional), vanilla extract and the psyllium to the beaten eggs and mix well with a fork.

4. Let the batter stand for 5-10 minutes so that it becomes a little stronger.

5. Heat a cast-iron poffertjes pan over high heat so that it becomes hot. Then grease the pan with a mild olive oil with a brush and lower the heat.

6. Now place a spoonful of batter in each compartment in the pan. Make sure you have lowered the heat now!

7. Bake the pancake for 2-4 minutes on one side (depending on how large the pancake is). When the top starts to dry, turn the poffertje with a spoon and bake the other side. Repeat until all the batter has been used up.

8. Beat the whipped cream with the vanilla extract or use a whipped cream machine.

9. Serve cold or hot.


Notes: Delicious with fresh raspberry or chia raspberry jam or chia blueberry jam or homemade keto-Nutella.

# Frittata with Chanterelles

## Nutrition

Calories: 1011 kcal | Gross carbohydrates: 13 g | Protein: 21 g | Fats: 97 g | Fiber: 4 g | Net carbohydrates: 9 g | Macro fats: 76 % | Macro proteins: 17 % | Macro carbohydrates: 7 %

Total time: 25 minutes

## Ingredients

6 eggs

250 grams of chanterelles

50 tablespoons butter

50 ml extra virgin olive oil

1 clove of garlic

1 tablespoon oregano leaves without stalk

1 tablespoon of young sage leaves

0.5 lemon

300 ml mascarpone

Creme fraiche dip

1 forest outing

200 ml creme fraiche

**Instructions**

1. Preheat the oven to 220° Celsius.

2. If the eggs are not yet at room temperature, remove them from the refrigerator and place them in a bowl of warm water (not boiling!).

3. Use a mushroom brush to gently clean the chanterelles. Leave them whole.

4. Heat the butter with the olive oil in a frying pan. Add the chanterelles to the pan as soon as the butter has melted and bake for 3-4 minutes until medium to high heat. Turn over occasionally.

5. Clean the garlic and chop it into small pieces.

6. Wash the sage and oregano, pat dry and chop into small pieces.

7. Add the garlic and spices to the skillet and turn the heat down. Cook for 4-5 minutes. Remove the pan from the heat and squeeze half a lemon over the chanterelles.

8. Grease a baking dish and / or put a sheet of baking paper in it.

9. Beat the eggs with the mascarpone in a bowl and add some salt and pepper.

10. Put the chanterelles in the baking dish and pour the beaten eggs over it. Bake in the oven for 10-15 minutes, until the egg is firm.

11. You can check whether the frittata is fully cooked by piercing it with a wooden or metal stick. If the skewer comes out clean, the frittata is ready.

12. Clean a spring onion and cut into rings. Mix through the creme fraiche.

13. Serve with creme fraiche.

# The Refreshing Nutter

Serving: 1

Prep Time: 10 minutes

**Ingredients:**

1 tablespoon chia seeds

2 cups water

1 ounces Macadamia Nuts

1-2 packets Stevia, optional

1 ounce hazelnut

**How To:**

1. Add all the listed ingredients to a blender.
2. Blend on high until smooth and creamy.
3. Enjoy your smoothie.

**Nutrition (Per Serving)**

Calories: 452

Fat: 43g

Carbohydrates: 15g

Protein: 9g

# Elegant Cranberry Muffins

Serving: 24 muffins

Prep Time: 10 minutes

Cooking Time: 20 minutes

**Ingredients:**

2 cups almond flour

2 teaspoons baking soda

¼ cup avocado oil

1 whole egg

¾ cup almond milk

½ cup Erythritol

½ cup apple sauce

Zest of 1 orange

2 teaspoons ground cinnamon

2 cup fresh cranberries

**How To:**

1. Pre-heat your oven to 350 degrees F.

2. Line muffin tin with paper muffin cups and keep them on the side.

3. Add flour, baking soda and keep it on the side.

4. Take another bowl and whisk in remaining ingredients and add flour, mix well.

5. Pour batter into prepared muffin tin and bake for 20 minutes.

6. Once done, let it cool for 10 minutes.

7. Serve and enjoy!

**Nutrition (Per Serving)**

Total Carbs: 7g

Fiber: 2g

Protein: 2.3g

Fat: 7g

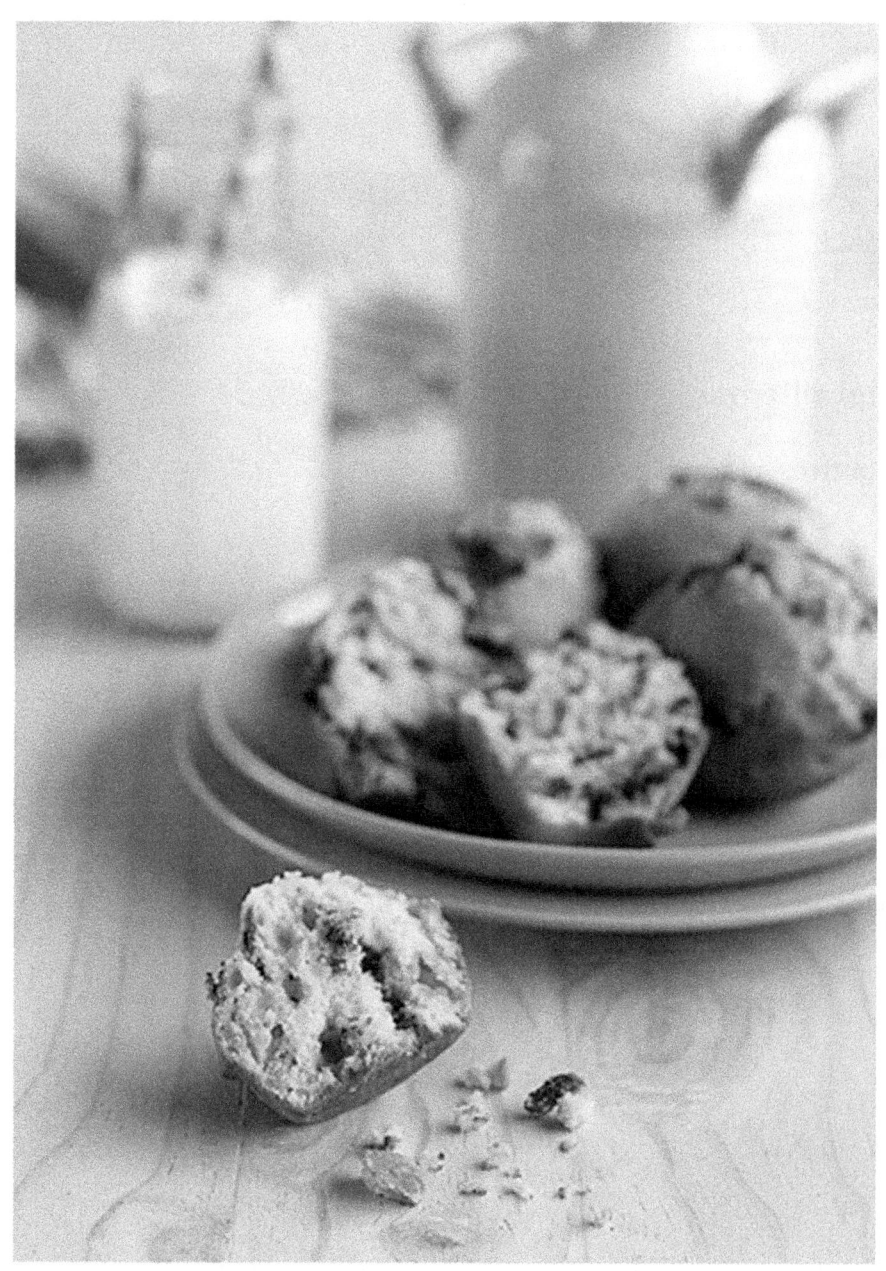

# Apple and Almond Muffins

Serving: 6 muffins

Prep Time: 10 minutes

Cooking Time: 20 minutes

**Ingredients:**

6 ounces ground almonds

1 teaspoon cinnamon

½ teaspoon baking powder

1 pinch sunflower seed

1 whole egg

1 teaspoon apple cider vinegar

2 tablespoons Erythritol

1/3 cup apple sauce

**How To:**

1. Pre-heat your oven to 350 degrees F.

2. Line muffin tin with paper muffin cups, keep them on the side.

3. Mix in almonds, cinnamon, baking powder, sunflower seeds and keep it on the side.

4. Take another bowl and beat in eggs, apple cider vinegar, apple sauce, Erythritol.

5. Add the mix to dry ingredients and mix well until you have a smooth batter.

6. Pour batter into tin and bake for 20 minutes.

7. Once done, let them cool.

8. Serve and enjoy!

**Nutrition (Per Serving)**

Total Carbs: 10

Fiber: 4g

Protein: 13g

Fat: 17g

# Stylish Chocolate Parfait

Serving: 4

Prep Time: 2 hours

Cook Time: nil

## Ingredients:

2 tablespoons cocoa powder

1 cup almond milk

1 tablespoon chia seeds

Pinch of sunflower seeds

½ teaspoon vanilla extract

## How To:

1. Take a bowl and add cocoa powder, almond milk, chia seeds, vanilla extract and stir.

2. Transfer to dessert glass and place in your fridge for 2 hours.

3. Serve and enjoy!

## Nutrition (Per Serving)

Calories: 130

Fat: 5g

Carbohydrates: 7g

Protein: 16g

# Supreme Matcha Bomb

Serving: 10

Prep Time: 100 minutes

Cook Time: Nil

**Ingredients:**

3/4 cup hemp seeds

½ cup coconut oil

2 tablespoons coconut almond butter

1 teaspoon Matcha powder

2 tablespoons vanilla bean extract

½ teaspoon mint extract Liquid stevia

**How To:**

1. Take your blender/food processor and add hemp seeds, coconut oil, Matcha, vanilla extract and stevia.

2. Blend until you have a nice batter and divide into silicon molds.

3. Melt coconut almond butter and drizzle on top.

4. Let the cups chill and enjoy!

**Nutrition (Per Serving)**

Calories: 200

Fat: 20g

Carbohydrates: 3g

Protein: 5g

# Mesmerizing Avocado and Chocolate Pudding

Serving: 2

Prep Time: 30 minutes

Cook Time: Nil

**Ingredients:**

1 avocado, chunked

1 tablespoon natural sweetener such as stevia

2 ounces cream cheese, at room temp

¼ teaspoon vanilla extract

4 tablespoons cocoa powder, unsweetened

**How To:**

1. Blend listed ingredients in blender until smooth.

2. Divide the mix between dessert bowls, chill for 30 minutes.

3. Serve and enjoy!

## Nutrition (Per Serving)

Calories: 281

Fat: 27g

Carbohydrates: 12g

Protein: 8g

# Hearty Pineapple Pudding

Serving: 4

Prep Time: 10 minutes

Cooking Time: 5 hours

**Ingredients:**

1 teaspoon baking powder

1 cup coconut flour

3 tablespoons stevia

3 tablespoons avocado oil

½ cup coconut milk

½ cup pecans, chopped

½ cup pineapple, chopped

½ cup lemon zest, grated

1 cup pineapple juice, natural

**How To:**

1. Grease Slow Cooker with oil.

2. Take a bowl and mix in flour, stevia, baking powder, oil, milk, pecans, pineapple, lemon zest, pineapple juice and stir well.

3. Pour the mix into the Slow Cooker.

4. Place lid and cook on LOW for 5 hours.

5. Divide between bowls and serve.

6. Enjoy!

**Nutrition (Per Serving)**

Calories: 188

Fat: 3g

Carbohydrates: 14g

Protein: 5g

# The Mean Green Smoothie

Serving: 2

Prep Time: 5 minutes

**Ingredients:**

1 avocado

1 handful spinach, chopped

Cucumber, 2 inch slices, peeled

1 lime, chopped

Handful of grapes, chopped

5 dates, stoned and chopped

1 cup apple juice (fresh)

**How To:**

1. Add all the listed ingredients to your blender.
2. Blend until smooth.
3. Add a few ice cubes and serve the smoothie.
4. Enjoy!

**Nutrition (Per Serving)**

Calories: 200

Fat: 10g

Carbohydrates: 14g

Protein 2g

# Mint Flavored Pear Smoothie

Serving: 2

Prep Time: 5 minutes

**Ingredients:**

¼ honey dew

2 green pears, ripe

½ apple, juiced 1 cup ice cubes

½ cup fresh mint leaves

**How To:**

Add the listed ingredients to your blender and blend until smooth. Serve chilled!

**Nutrition (Per Serving)**

Calories: 200

Fat: 10g

Carbohydrates: 14g

Protein 2g

# Chilled Watermelon Smoothie

Serving: 2

Prep Time: 5 minutes

**Ingredients:**

1 cup watermelon chunks

½ cup coconut water

1 ½ teaspoons lime juice

4 mint leaves

4 ice cubes

**How To:**

1. Add the listed ingredients to your blender and blend until smooth.

2. Serve chilled!

## Nutrition (Per Serving)

Calories: 200

Fat: 10g

Carbohydrates: 14g

Protein 2g

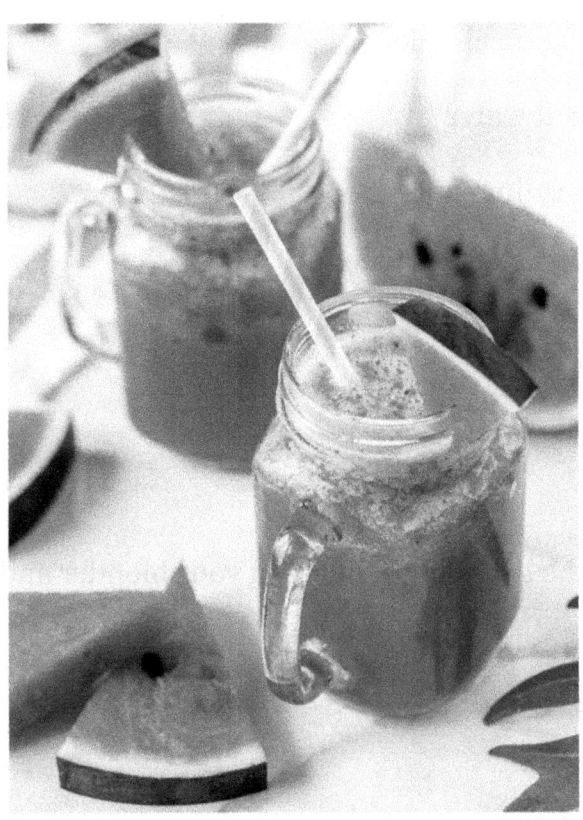

# Banana Ginger Medley

Serving: 2

Prep Time: 5 minutes

**Ingredients:**

1 banana, sliced

¾ cup vanilla yogurt

1 tablespoon honey

½ teaspoon ginger, grated

**How To:**

1. Add the listed ingredients to your blender and blend until smooth.

2. Serve chilled!

**Nutrition (Per Serving)**

Calories: 200
Fat: 10g
Carbohydrates: 14g
Protein 2g

# Banana and Almond Flax Glass

Serving: 2

Prep Time: 5 minutes

**Ingredients:**

1 ripe frozen banana, diced

2/3 cup unsweetened almond milk

1/3 cup fat free plain Greek Yogurt

1 ½ tablespoons almond butter

1 tablespoon flaxseed meal

1 teaspoon honey

2-3 drops almond extract

**How To:**

Add the listed ingredients to your blender and blend until smooth Serve chilled!

**Nutrition (Per Serving)**

Calories: 200

Fat: 10g

Carbohydrates: 14g

## Protein 2g

# Spicy Wasabi Mayonnaise

Serving: 4

Prep Time: 15 minutes

Cook Time: Nil

## Ingredients:

1 cup mayonnaise

½ tablespoon wasabi paste

## How To:

1. Take a bowl and mix wasabi paste and mayonnaise.
2. Mix well.
3. Let it chill and use as needed.

## Nutrition (Per Serving)

Calories: 388

Fat: 42g

Carbohydrates: 1g

Protein: 1g

# Mediterranean Kale Dish

Serving: 6

Prep Time: 15 minutes

Cook Time: 10 minutes

## Ingredients:

12 cups kale, chopped

2 tablespoons lemon juice

1 tablespoon olive oil

1 teaspoon coconut aminos

Sunflower seeds and pepper as needed

## How To:

1. Add a steamer insert to your saucepan.

2. Fill the saucepan with water up to the bottom of the steamer.

3. Cover and bring water to boil (medium-high heat).

4. Add kale to the insert and steam for 7-8 minutes.

5. Take a large bowl and add lemon juice, olive oil, sunflower seeds, coconut aminos, and pepper.

6. Mix well and add the steamed kale to the bowl.

7. Toss and serve.

8. Enjoy!

**Nutrition (Per Serving)**

Calories: 350

Fat: 17g

Carbohydrates: 41g

Protein: 11g

# Delicious Garlic Tomatoes

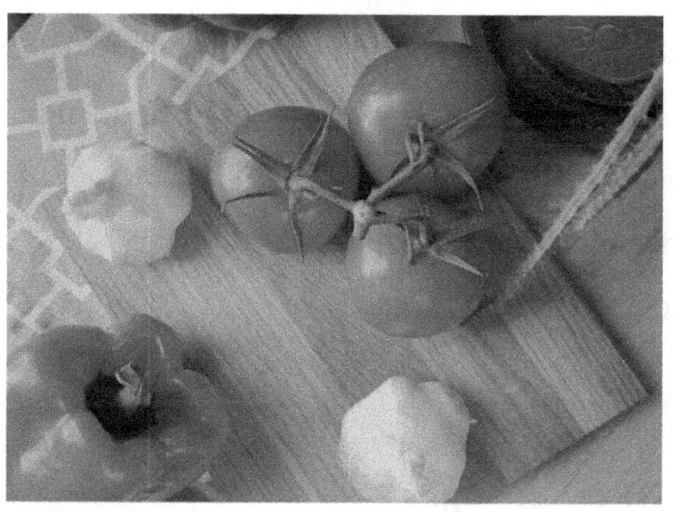

Serving: 4

Prep Time: 10 minutes

Cook Time: 50 minutes

**Ingredients:**

4 garlic cloves, crushed

1 pound mixed cherry tomatoes

3 thyme sprigs, chopped

Pinch of sunflower seeds

Black pepper as needed

¼ cup olive oil

**How To:**

1. Preheat your oven to 325 degrees F.
2. Take a baking dish and add tomatoes, olive oil and thyme.
3. Season with sunflower seeds and pepper and mix.
4. Bake for 50 minutes.
5. Divide tomatoes and pan juices and serve.
6. Enjoy!

**Nutrition (Per Serving)**

Calories: 100

Fat: 0g

Carbohydrates: 1g

Protein: 6g

# Mashed Celeriac

Serving: 4

Prep Time: 10 minutes

Cook Time: 20 minutes

**Ingredients:**

2 celeriac, washed, peeled and diced

2 teaspoons extra-virgin olive oil

1 tablespoon honey

½ teaspoon ground nutmeg

Sunflower seeds and pepper as needed

**How To:**

1. Pre-heat your oven to 400 degrees F.
2. Line a baking sheet with aluminum foil and keep it on the side.
3. Take a large bowl and toss celeriac and olive oil.
4. Spread celeriac evenly on a baking sheet.
5. Roast for 20 minutes until tender.
6. Transfer to a large bowl.
7. Add honey and nutmeg.
8. Use a potato masher to mash the mixture until fluffy.

9. Season with sunflower seeds and pepper.

10. Serve and enjoy!

**Nutrition (Per Serving)**

Calories: 136

Fat: 3g

Carbohydrates: 26g

Protein: 4g

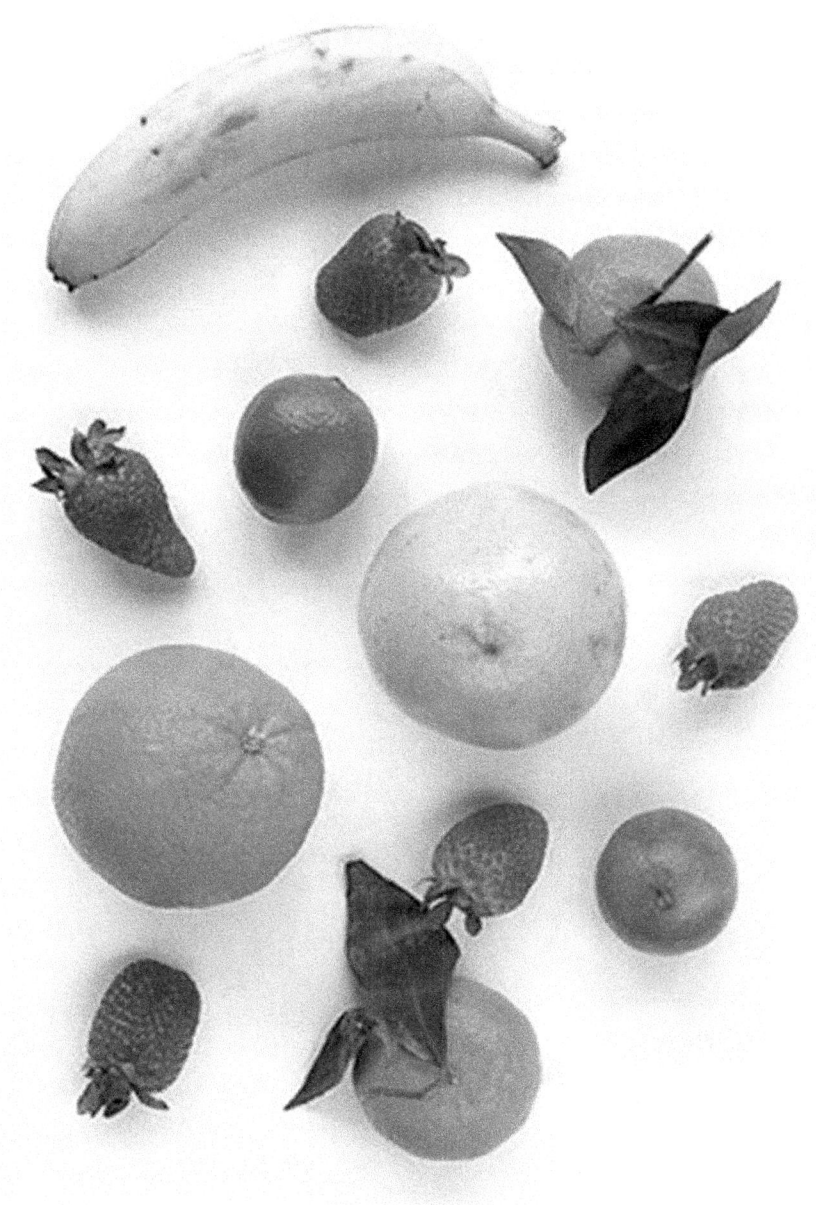

www.ingramcontent.com/pod-product-compliance
Lightning Source LLC
Chambersburg PA
CBHW071109030426
42336CB00013BA/2017